WEIGHT LOSS SMOOTHIES

Transform Your Health, Boost Energy, and Achieve Your Ideal Weight

Karen Brown

Table of Contents

INTRODUCTION

A Delicious Path To Transformation

Welcome to the tantalising world of weight loss smoothies—a delicious path to transformation that will not only help you shed unwanted pounds but also tantalise your taste buds along the way. Gone are the days of restrictive diets and flavourless meals; instead, we invite you to embark on a culinary adventure that will redefine your perception of healthy eating. In this journey, we will explore the art of crafting weight loss smoothies that are not only nourishing but also delightful to the senses. Get ready to savour vibrant flavours, indulge in nutritious ingredients, and witness the transformative power of these delectable beverages. So, grab your blender and join us as we embark on a mouthwatering voyage towards a healthier and happier you. This is the delicious path to transformation for weight loss smoothies.

CHAPTER ONE

Understanding The Science Behind Weight Loss Smoothies

The Role of Macronutrients in Weight Loss

When it comes to weight loss, one cannot overlook the crucial role that macronutrients play in achieving and maintaining a healthy body weight. Macronutrients, also known as "macros," are the essential nutrients that our bodies require in large quantities: carbohydrates, proteins, and fats. Understanding the impact of these macronutrients on weight loss can empower individuals to make informed dietary choices and embark on a successful weight management journey.

Carbohydrates: Carbs have often been vilified in popular weight loss trends, but they are an important energy source for our bodies. Complex carbohydrates, found in whole grains, legumes, fruits, and vegetables, provide sustained energy and essential fiber. They are a vital component of a balanced diet and can aid weight loss by promoting satiety and preventing overeating. It's crucial to focus on consuming whole, unprocessed carbohydrates and avoid excessive intake of refined sugars and processed foods.

Proteins: Protein is an invaluable macronutrient when it comes to weight loss.

It supports the growth and repair of tissues, aids in muscle development, and helps maintain a feeling of fullness. Including lean sources of protein such as poultry, fish, tofu, beans, and Greek yoghurt in your diet can contribute to increased satiety, reduced calorie intake, and improved body composition. Protein also has a higher thermic effect, meaning it requires more energy to digest and metabolise, potentially boosting calorie expenditure.

Fats: Dietary fat is often misunderstood as a contributor to weight gain, but not all fats are created equal. Healthy fats, such as those found in avocados, nuts, seeds, and olive oil, are essential for overall well-being and weight management. Including moderate amounts of healthy fats in your diet can enhance satiety, support hormone production, and aid in the absorption of fat-soluble vitamins. However, it's essential to practise portion control, as fats are calorie-dense.

Choosing the Right Ingredients for Maximum Results

When it comes to crafting weight loss smoothies, choosing the right ingredients is key to achieving maximum results. By incorporating nutrient-dense and metabolism-boosting ingredients, you can create smoothies that not only support your weight loss goals but also provide a satisfying and delicious experience. Let's explore the essential components for creating smoothies that deliver maximum results on your weight loss journey.

Fibre-Rich Fruits and Vegetables: Incorporating fibre into your smoothies is crucial for promoting satiety and maintaining steady blood sugar levels. Opt for low-glycemic fruits such as berries, apples, and pears, which are rich in antioxidants and fibre. Leafy greens like spinach and kale are also excellent additions, as they are low in calories and packed with essential vitamins and minerals.

Protein Powerhouses: Protein is a macronutrient that aids in muscle recovery, promotes a feeling of fullness, and supports a healthy metabolism. Adding a high-quality protein source to your smoothies, such as Greek yoghourt, cottage cheese, or a plant-based protein powder, can help control cravings and maintain muscle mass during weight loss.

Healthy Fats: While it may seem counterintuitive, including healthy fats in your weight loss smoothies can be beneficial. Fats provide a sense of satiety, slow down digestion, and help absorb fat-soluble vitamins. Avocado, almond butter, chia seeds, and flaxseeds are excellent choices to incorporate healthy fats and add creaminess to your smoothies.

Metabolism-Boosting Additions: Certain ingredients can help rev up your metabolism and enhance the fat-burning potential of your smoothies. Consider adding metabolism-boosting spices like cinnamon or cayenne pepper, green tea extract, or ginger to provide an extra kick. These ingredients may increase thermogenesis, leading to a temporary rise in calorie expenditure.

Hydration and Liquid Choices: Staying hydrated is essential for overall health and weight management. Incorporate hydrating ingredients like coconut water or unsweetened almond milk as the liquid base for your smoothies. Avoid sugary juices or sweetened dairy products, as they can add unnecessary calories.

Mindful Sweeteners: While it's best to limit added sugars, a touch of natural sweetness can enhance the flavour of your smoothies. Opt for natural sweeteners such as raw honey, pure maple syrup, or dates, but use them sparingly to avoid excessive calorie intake.

Blending Techniques for Optimal Nutrition

Blending techniques play a crucial role in maximising the nutritional benefits of weight loss smoothies. By employing the right methods, you can ensure that your smoothies retain their nutrient content, achieve a desirable texture, and enhance the absorption of key ingredients. Let's explore some blending techniques that will help you optimise the nutrition of your weight loss smoothies.

Start with a Solid Foundation: Begin by adding the liquid component, such as water, unsweetened almond milk, or coconut water, to the blender. This will provide a base for your smoothie and help the ingredients blend smoothly.

Layer Ingredients Wisely: Layering ingredients in the blender can make the blending process more efficient. Start with the bulkier ingredients like leafy greens, followed by softer fruits, proteins, healthy fats, and any powders or spices. This layering technique ensures even blending and prevents ingredients from getting stuck at the bottom.

Gradually Increase Speed: When blending, start at a low speed and gradually increase to higher speeds. This approach helps break down the ingredients evenly and prevents over-blending, which can lead to a loss of nutrients and a less desirable texture.

Blend Until Smooth: Aim to blend your smoothie until it reaches a smooth and creamy consistency. This ensures that all the ingredients are well incorporated and maximises the bioavailability of nutrients.

Use Short Bursts and Pulsing: For smoother blending, employ short bursts or pulsing techniques. This helps dislodge any stubborn pieces or chunks, ensuring a more consistent texture.

Add Ice Last: If you prefer a chilled smoothie, add ice cubes as the final step. This prevents the smoothie from becoming too diluted and maintains its thickness and flavour.

Consume Immediately or Store Properly: To retain the optimal nutrition of your smoothie, consume it immediately after blending. If you need to store it for later, place it in an airtight container and refrigerate. However, note that some nutrient degradation may occur over time, so it's best to consume it within a day or two.

Experiment with Blending Times: Depending on the ingredients you use, you may want to experiment with blending times. Some ingredients, like leafy greens, may require a longer blending duration to break down completely. Adjusting the blending time can help you achieve the desired consistency and maximise nutrient release.

CHAPTER TWO

Preparing Your Kitchen for Smoothie Success

Essential Tools and Equipment

To embark on your weight loss smoothie journey with ease and efficiency, it's important to have the right tools and equipment at your disposal. These essential tools will not only simplify the process of preparing your smoothies but also contribute to their quality and enjoyment. Let's explore the must-have tools and equipment for crafting delicious and nutritious weight loss smoothies.

High-Quality Blender: A high-quality blender is the cornerstone of smoothie preparation. Look for a blender with a powerful motor, sturdy construction, and sharp blades. A blender with variable speeds and different blending settings can provide greater control over the texture of your smoothies. Whether you choose a countertop blender or a personal blender, invest in a model that meets your specific needs and budget.

Measuring Tools: Accurate measurements are crucial when it comes to portion control and maintaining the desired nutritional balance in your smoothies. Having measuring cups and spoons on hand allows you to precisely measure your ingredients, ensuring consistency and tracking calorie intake.

Cutting Board and Knife: A reliable cutting board and a sharp knife are essential for preparing fruits, vegetables, and other ingredients. They facilitate efficient and safe chopping, dicing, and slicing, enabling you to quickly and easily prepare your smoothie ingredients.

Mason Jars or Portable Bottles: Having mason jars or portable bottles with tight-sealing lids is convenient for storing and transporting your smoothies. These containers help maintain freshness and prevent leaks, allowing you to enjoy your smoothies on the go or prepare them in advance for a busy day.

Ice Cube Trays: Ice cubes can add a refreshing touch to your smoothies while maintaining their thickness. Using ice cube trays allows you to freeze ingredients like coconut water, almond milk, or blended fruits for quick and easy additions to your smoothies.

Cleaning Tools: Keeping your tools and equipment clean is essential for hygiene and maintaining the integrity of your smoothies. Have a bottle brush, dishcloth, or sponge dedicated to cleaning your blender and other utensils. Additionally, a dishwasher-safe blender is a convenient option for easy cleanup.

Stocking Your Pantry and Fridge

Stocking your pantry and fridge with the right ingredients is key to ensuring you have a wide array of nutritious options for your weight loss smoothies. By keeping a well-stocked selection of ingredients, you'll be able to create delicious and satisfying smoothies while staying on track with your health goals. Here are some essential items to consider adding to your pantry and fridge for weight loss smoothies:

Fruits: Keep a variety of fresh and frozen fruits on hand. Opt for low-glycemic options such as berries (strawberries, blueberries, raspberries), apples, pears, and citrus fruits. These fruits are packed with vitamins, antioxidants, and fibre, while being relatively low in calories and sugar.

Leafy Greens: Include nutrient-dense leafy greens such as spinach, kale, and Swiss chard. These greens are low in calories and high in vitamins, minerals, and fibre. Adding a handful of greens to your smoothies boosts their nutritional value without compromising flavour.

Protein Sources: Have a selection of protein sources available, such as Greek yoghurt, cottage cheese, tofu, or plant-based protein powders. Protein helps promote satiety, supports muscle recovery, and aids in weight management.

Healthy Fats: Include sources of healthy fats in your pantry and fridge, such as avocados, nuts (almonds, walnuts), seeds (chia seeds, flaxseeds), and nut butters (almond butter, peanut butter). These ingredients provide satiety, essential fatty acids, and a creamy texture to your smoothies.

Liquid Bases: Stock up on liquid bases like unsweetened almond milk, coconut water, or low-fat dairy milk (if preferred). These provide a smooth consistency to your smoothies while keeping them hydrated and flavorful.

Spices and Additives: Have a collection of spices and additives to enhance the flavour and nutritional profile of your smoothies. Consider cinnamon, ginger, turmeric, cocoa powder, or matcha powder. These ingredients add depth and a metabolic boost to your smoothies.

Freezer Staples: Keep your freezer stocked with frozen fruits, such as berries, mangoes, and pineapple. These serve as a convenient way to add a frosty element to your smoothies while extending their shelf life. You can also freeze coconut water or almond milk in ice cube trays for easy blending.

Tips for Organizing Smoothie Ingredients

Organising your smoothie ingredients is a helpful strategy to streamline your preparation process and ensure that you have everything you need at your fingertips. By establishing an organised system, you can save time, minimise waste, and maintain a well-stocked supply of ingredients for your weight loss smoothies. Here are some tips to help you organise your smoothie ingredients effectively:

Designate a Smoothie Station: Set aside a dedicated area in your kitchen as your "smoothie station." This can be a countertop or a designated shelf in your pantry or fridge. Having a designated space will make it easier to keep track of your smoothie ingredients and prevent them from getting mixed up with other items.

Categorise Ingredients: Group your smoothie ingredients into categories based on their type or purpose. For example, create separate sections for fruits, leafy greens, protein sources, healthy fats, spices, and sweeteners. This categorization makes it easier to locate specific ingredients when preparing your smoothies.

Use Clear Containers: Store your ingredients in clear, airtight containers to keep them visible and fresh. Mason jars, clear plastic bins, or glass containers are great options. Label the containers if needed, especially if you have multiple containers with similar-looking ingredients.

Prioritise Accessibility: Arrange your ingredients in a way that promotes easy access. Place frequently used items within arm's reach or at eye level. Reserve the lower shelves or drawers for larger or less frequently used items.

Create a FIFO System: FIFO stands for "First In, First Out." To avoid ingredient spoilage, practice rotating your stock by placing newly purchased items behind older ones. This ensures that you use the older ingredients first and reduces the chances of forgetting about certain items.

Invest in Storage Solutions: Consider investing in storage solutions that maximise space utilisation and keep your ingredients organised. Options include stacking bins, lazy susans, drawer dividers, or tiered shelves. These tools can help optimise your storage capacity and make ingredient retrieval more efficient.

Take Inventory Regularly: Set aside time to take inventory of your smoothie ingredients on a regular basis. Check expiration dates, discard any expired items, and make note of ingredients that need replenishing. This practice helps you maintain a well-stocked pantry and fridge, reducing the likelihood of running out of essential ingredients.

Plan and Prep Ahead: Consider prepping your ingredients in advance to save time during busy mornings. Wash and chop your fruits and vegetables, portion out your protein sources, and prepare any homemade blends or spice mixes. Store them in individual containers or freezer bags for easy use when making your smoothies.

CHAPTER THREE

Energising Morning Smoothies

Rise and Shine: Breakfast Boosters

Starting your day with a nutritious and satisfying breakfast is essential, especially when you're on a weight loss journey. Weight loss smoothies can be a fantastic option for breakfast, providing a convenient and delicious way to fuel your body and kick-start your metabolism. To give your weight loss smoothies an extra boost, incorporate these breakfast boosters that will help you stay energised, satisfied, and on track with your goals.

Oats: Adding oats to your weight loss smoothies provides a good dose of fibre and complex carbohydrates, which promote feelings of fullness and provide sustained energy throughout the morning. Use rolled oats or quick oats, and blend them into your smoothie for added texture and thickness.

Greek Yoghourt: Greek yoghourt is a protein-rich ingredient that adds creaminess and tanginess to your smoothies. It not only provides a good source of protein but also contains probiotics that support gut health. Choose plain, unsweetened Greek yoghurt to keep added sugars in check.

Nut Butter: Incorporating a spoonful of nut butter, such as almond butter or peanut butter, into your smoothies adds healthy fats, protein, and a rich, nutty flavour. Nut butter can help increase satiety, promote a feeling of fullness, and add a velvety texture to your smoothies.

Chia Seeds: Chia seeds are tiny nutritional powerhouses packed with fibre, omega-3 fatty acids, and antioxidants. When added to your smoothies, they absorb liquid and create a thick and satisfying texture. Chia seeds also help regulate blood sugar levels and promote digestive health.

Flaxseeds: Flaxseeds are another excellent addition to boost the nutritional value of your smoothies. They are rich in omega-3 fatty acids, fibre, and lignans, which have antioxidant properties. Grind flax seeds before adding them to your smoothies to enhance their digestibility and maximise nutrient absorption.

Berries: Berries, such as strawberries, blueberries, raspberries, and blackberries, are not only delicious but also low in calories and high in antioxidants and fibre. They add natural sweetness, vibrant colour, and a burst of flavour to your weight loss smoothies without significantly increasing the calorie content.

Greens: Don't shy away from adding leafy greens like spinach, kale, or Swiss chard to your breakfast smoothies. They are packed with essential vitamins, minerals, and fibre while being low in calories. The mild taste of leafy greens blends well with other ingredients, ensuring you get a nutrient-packed start to your day.

Unsweetened Almond Milk: Using unsweetened almond milk as the liquid base for your smoothies provides a creamy texture without adding excessive calories or sugar. It's a good alternative for those who are lactose intolerant or following a dairy-free lifestyle.

Metabolism Kickstarters

If you're looking to give your weight loss efforts a boost, incorporating metabolism kickstarters into your smoothies can be a game-changer. These ingredients are known for their ability to rev up your metabolism, increase calorie burn, and support your weight loss goals. By adding these metabolism-boosting ingredients to your weight loss smoothies, you can supercharge your efforts and enhance your body's fat-burning potential. Here are some key metabolism kickstarters to consider:

Green Tea: Green tea contains catechins, which are powerful antioxidants known for their metabolism-boosting properties. Brew a cup of green tea and allow it to cool before using it as the liquid base for your smoothie. Alternatively, you can add matcha powder, which is made from ground green tea leaves, directly to your smoothie.

Cayenne Pepper: Cayenne pepper contains a compound called capsaicin, which has thermogenic properties.

Thermogenesis is the process by which your body generates heat and burns calories. Adding a pinch of cayenne pepper to your smoothie can increase your metabolism and enhance fat burning.

Cinnamon: Cinnamon is not only a delicious spice but also a metabolism booster. It helps regulate blood sugar levels, which in turn can stabilise insulin levels and support weight loss efforts. Sprinkle a teaspoon of cinnamon into your smoothie to enjoy its metabolism-boosting benefits.

Ginger: Ginger has long been known for its digestive and metabolism-boosting properties. It can increase calorie burn and improve the absorption of nutrients. Add a small piece of fresh ginger or a teaspoon of ginger powder to your smoothies for a zesty kick and metabolic support.

Coconut Oil: Coconut oil contains medium-chain triglycerides (MCTs), which are easily absorbed and used as a quick source of energy by the body. MCTs can boost your metabolism and promote fat burning. Add a tablespoon of coconut oil to your smoothies to enjoy its metabolic benefits.

Apple Cider Vinegar: Apple cider vinegar has been shown to improve insulin sensitivity and reduce blood sugar levels. These effects can support weight loss efforts and enhance metabolism. Incorporate a tablespoon of apple cider vinegar into your smoothies for its metabolic benefits. Be mindful of its strong taste and start with smaller amounts.

Protein-Rich Ingredients: Protein requires more energy to digest compared to fats and carbohydrates, which means it can temporarily boost your metabolism. Include protein-rich ingredients like Greek yoghurt, tofu, or protein powder in your smoothies to promote muscle growth, increase satiety, and support metabolic function.

High-Fibre Ingredients: High-fibre foods, such as chia seeds, flaxseeds, and leafy greens, can help boost metabolism by promoting fullness and regulating digestion. Fibre also requires more energy to break down, which can further support calorie burn. Add these fibre-rich ingredients to your weight loss smoothies for added metabolic benefits.

Supercharge Your Mornings with Protein

To supercharge your mornings and support your weight loss goals, incorporating protein into your smoothies is a fantastic strategy. Protein is a macronutrient that plays a crucial role in building and repairing tissues, supporting muscle growth, and promoting feelings of satiety. By adding protein to your weight loss smoothies, you can enhance their nutritional value, increase fullness, and support your body's fat-burning potential. Here's why protein is important and how you can supercharge your mornings with protein-packed weight loss smoothies:

Promotes Satiety: Protein is known to be more satisfying and filling compared to carbohydrates and fats. Including protein in your smoothies can help curb cravings and keep you feeling satisfied for longer, reducing the likelihood of overeating later in the day.

Supports Muscle Development: Protein is essential for muscle repair and growth. Including protein in your breakfast smoothies can help preserve and build lean muscle mass, which is important for maintaining a healthy metabolism. As you increase your muscle mass, your body becomes more efficient at burning calories, even at rest.

Enhances Metabolism: Protein has a higher thermic effect of food (TEF) compared to carbohydrates and fats, which means that your body burns more calories during digestion and absorption. By incorporating protein into your weight loss smoothies, you can give your metabolism a boost and increase calorie burn.

Stabilises Blood Sugar Levels: Protein can help slow down the absorption of sugar into the bloodstream, preventing spikes and crashes in blood sugar levels. This can help regulate your energy levels throughout the morning and reduce cravings for unhealthy snacks.

Now, let's explore some protein-rich ingredients that you can add to your weight loss smoothies:

Cottage Cheese: Cottage cheese is another protein powerhouse that blends well in smoothies. It provides a creamy texture and adds a boost of protein without adding excessive calories.

Silken Tofu: Silken tofu is a plant-based protein option that works well in smoothies. It has a smooth and creamy texture and can be a great alternative for those following a vegetarian or vegan lifestyle.

Protein Powder: Protein powder, such as whey, soy, or plant-based varieties, can be a convenient option to increase protein content in your smoothies. Choose a high-quality protein powder without added sugars or artificial ingredients.

Nut Butter: Nut butter, such as almond butter or peanut butter, not only adds protein but also provides healthy fats and a rich, creamy flavour to your smoothies. Ensure you choose natural nut butters without added sugars or hydrogenated oils.

Hemp Seeds: Hemp seeds are a plant-based protein source that contains all essential amino acids. They add a nutty flavour and a nutritional boost to your smoothies.

CHAPTER FOUR

Satisfying Meal Replacement Smoothies

Fulfilling and Nutrient-Packed Lunch Options

When it comes to weight loss, lunchtime offers a fantastic opportunity to refuel your body with fulfilling and nutrient-packed meals. While weight loss smoothies are a popular choice for breakfast, there are plenty of other options to consider for a satisfying midday meal. These lunch options not only support your weight loss goals but also provide a range of nutrients to keep you energised throughout the day. Here are some fulfilling and nutrient-packed lunch ideas to complement your weight loss journey:

Colourful Salad Bowls: Create a vibrant and filling salad by combining a variety of leafy greens, colourful vegetables, lean protein sources, and healthy fats. Consider adding ingredients like grilled chicken or turkey, boiled eggs, chickpeas, avocado, nuts, seeds, and a homemade dressing made with olive oil and vinegar or lemon juice.

Veggie Wraps or Collard Green Wraps: Wrap up a flavorful combination of fresh veggies, lean protein, and whole-grain wraps or collard green leaves. Fill them with ingredients like grilled tofu, tempeh, sliced turkey or chicken breast, mixed greens, tomatoes, cucumbers, sprouts, and a light spread of hummus or mashed avocado.

Quinoa or Brown Rice Bowls: Build a satisfying bowl by combining cooked quinoa or brown rice with a variety of veggies, protein, and healthy fats. Top it with grilled shrimp, chicken, or tofu, and add roasted vegetables, steamed greens, sliced avocado, and a sprinkle of herbs and spices for flavour.

Soup and Salad Combo: Enjoy a hearty and nourishing soup paired with a side salad for a well-rounded lunch. Opt for homemade soups made with lean proteins like chicken, turkey, or lentils, combined with a variety of vegetables. Pair it with a salad featuring mixed greens, cherry tomatoes, cucumber, carrots, and a light dressing.

Protein-Packed Sandwiches or Wraps: Choose whole-grain bread or wraps and fill them with lean protein sources like turkey, chicken, grilled fish, or plant-based options such as tofu or tempeh. Add a variety of vegetables like lettuce, tomato, cucumber, and sprouts, and use a light spread like mustard or hummus for flavour.

Buddha Bowls: Assemble a nourishing Buddha bowl with a combination of cooked grains (quinoa, brown rice, or farro), roasted or sautéed vegetables, a protein source like grilled chicken, tofu, or beans, and a drizzle of a homemade dressing or sauce.

Stir-Fries: Create a quick and healthy stir-fry by sautéing a mix of colourful vegetables like broccoli, bell peppers, carrots, snap peas, and mushrooms. Add lean proteins such as shrimp, chicken, or tofu, and season with soy sauce, ginger, and garlic. Serve it over cauliflower rice or brown rice for a fulfilling meal.

Protein-Packed Soups: Opt for protein-rich soups like lentil soup, chicken vegetable soup, or black bean soup. These soups provide a balance of nutrients, including fibre, protein, and a variety of vegetables, keeping you satisfied throughout the afternoon.

Savory and Filling Dinner Smoothies

When it comes to dinner, smoothies may not be the first thing that comes to mind. However, savoury and filling dinner smoothies can be a nutritious and convenient option for those seeking a lighter and refreshing meal in the evening. These dinner smoothies can incorporate a variety of vegetables, proteins, and healthy fats to create a satisfying and balanced meal. Here are some ideas for creating savoury and filling dinner smoothies:

Green Vegetable Powerhouse: Blend together a combination of leafy greens like spinach or kale, cucumber, celery, avocado, and herbs such as parsley or cilantro. Add a scoop of protein powder, a splash of vegetable broth or almond milk, and season with spices like garlic powder, cayenne pepper, or sea salt for added flavour.

Creamy Tomato Basil: Combine tomatoes, roasted red peppers, fresh basil leaves, Greek yoghourt or silken tofu, and a dash of olive oil in a blender. Season with salt, pepper, and Italian seasoning to taste. This smoothie is reminiscent of a creamy tomato soup and can be served warm or chilled.

Mexican-Inspired Black Bean: Blend together cooked black beans, diced tomatoes, bell peppers, red onion, cilantro, lime juice, and a dash of cumin and chilli powder. You can also add a small avocado or a spoonful of Greek yoghourt for creaminess. Serve with a sprinkle of shredded cheese or tortilla strips on top.

Mediterranean Delight: Create a smoothie with a Mediterranean twist by combining roasted red bell peppers, cucumber, Kalamata olives, artichoke hearts, feta cheese, lemon juice, and a drizzle of extra virgin olive oil. Add a handful of fresh herbs like parsley or mint for added freshness.

Enhancing Satiety with Fiber-Rich Ingredients

If you're looking to enhance satiety and support your weight loss goals, incorporating fibre-rich ingredients into your smoothies is a smart strategy. Fibre is a type of carbohydrate that is not digested by the body, which means it adds bulk to your diet without contributing calories. Fibre-rich foods help you feel full and satisfied, reducing the likelihood of overeating and promoting weight loss. Here's how you can enhance satiety with fibre-rich ingredients in your weight loss smoothies:

Leafy Greens: Add a handful of spinach, kale, or Swiss chard to your smoothies. These greens are low in calories and high in fibre, making them an excellent addition for boosting satiety. They also offer a range of vitamins, minerals, and antioxidants.

Chia Seeds: Chia seeds are a nutritional powerhouse, packed with fibre and omega-3 fatty acids. They have the ability to absorb liquid and form a gel-like consistency, which can help keep you feeling full for longer. Add a tablespoon of chia seeds to your smoothie and allow them to soak for a few minutes before consuming.

Berries: Berries like raspberries, blackberries, strawberries, and blueberries are not only delicious but also high in fibre. They add natural sweetness and antioxidants to your smoothies while boosting their fibre content.

Avocado: Avocado is a creamy and nutrient-rich fruit that is high in fibre and healthy monounsaturated fats. It adds a smooth and velvety texture to your smoothies while helping to keep you full and satisfied.

Beans and Legumes: Consider adding cooked beans or legumes like chickpeas, black beans, or lentils to your smoothies. They are excellent sources of both fibre and plant-based protein, making them a satisfying addition to your weight loss smoothies.

CHAPTER FIVE

Post-Workout and Recovery Smoothies

Replenishing Nutrients after Exercise

After exercise, it's crucial to replenish your body with the necessary nutrients to support recovery and aid in weight loss. One effective way to accomplish this is by incorporating nutrient-rich smoothies into your post-workout routine. These smoothies provide a convenient and easily digestible source of essential vitamins, minerals, and macronutrients. Here are some key components to consider when creating replenishing weight loss smoothies after exercise:

Hydration: Rehydration is a top priority after any workout. Start by including a liquid base in your smoothie such as water, coconut water, or unsweetened almond milk. These options help replenish fluids lost through sweat and support optimal hydration.

Protein Power: Protein is crucial for muscle repair and recovery after exercise. Include a high-quality protein source in your smoothie, such as Greek yoghourt, whey protein powder, or plant-based options like pea or hemp protein. Aim for around 20-30 grams of protein per serving.

Antioxidant Boost: Exercise can generate oxidative stress in the body, so adding antioxidant-rich ingredients like berries (blueberries, strawberries), dark leafy greens, or matcha green tea powder can help counteract free radicals and promote overall recovery.

Electrolyte Balancing: Sweating during exercise leads to the loss of electrolytes like sodium, potassium, and magnesium. Replace these vital minerals by incorporating ingredients like coconut water, a pinch of sea salt, or electrolyte-rich fruits such as bananas or oranges.

Optional Supplements: Depending on your specific needs, you may consider adding supplements like collagen powder for joint health, spirulina for an additional boost of nutrients, or turmeric for its anti-inflammatory properties. Consult with a physician to determine which supplements are suitable for you.

Muscle Recovery and Repair Boosters

Muscle recovery and repair are essential aspects of any fitness regimen, and incorporating specific ingredients into your weight loss smoothies can provide a boost to these processes. These ingredients support muscle recovery by providing essential nutrients that aid in repairing damaged muscle tissue and reducing inflammation. Here are some muscle recovery and repair boosters to consider when creating weight loss smoothies:

Tart Cherry Juice: Tart cherry juice has been shown to possess anti-inflammatory properties and aid in reducing muscle soreness. Its natural antioxidants, specifically anthocyanins, may help speed up muscle recovery. Add a splash of tart cherry juice to your smoothie for a tart and refreshing twist.

Leafy Greens: Dark leafy greens like spinach and kale are packed with nutrients such as iron, calcium, and vitamins A and C. These nutrients are essential for muscle repair and can help reduce inflammation. Add a handful of greens to your smoothie for an extra nutritional boost.

Omega-3 Fatty Acids: Omega-3 fatty acids have been shown to possess anti-inflammatory properties and support muscle recovery. Add a tablespoon of ground flaxseeds, chia seeds, or a teaspoon of fish oil to your smoothie to provide a dose of these healthy fats.

Coconut Water: Coconut water is a natural source of electrolytes like potassium and magnesium, which are important for muscle function and recovery. Including coconut water as the liquid base for your smoothie helps replenish electrolytes lost during exercise.

Natural Yoghourt or Kefir: Natural yoghourt or kefir contains probiotics, which promote a healthy gut environment. A healthy gut can enhance nutrient absorption, support immune function, and aid in overall recovery. Add a scoop of natural yoghourt or kefir to your smoothie for a creamy and probiotic-rich addition.

Hydration and Electrolyte Imbalances

Hydration and electrolyte balance are key factors in maintaining optimal health, especially during weight loss and exercise. When creating weight loss smoothies, incorporating ingredients that hydrate and replenish electrolytes can be beneficial for overall well-being. Here are some hydration and electrolyte rebalancers to consider when making your weight loss smoothies:

Watermelon: Watermelon is not only delicious but also incredibly hydrating due to its high water content. It also contains natural electrolytes like potassium, making it an excellent choice for refreshing smoothies.

Cucumber: Cucumber is another hydrating ingredient that adds a refreshing taste to your smoothies. It is rich in water, providing hydration, and contains minerals like potassium and magnesium, which help maintain electrolyte balance.

Aloe Vera Juice: Aloe vera juice is known for its hydrating properties and can help soothe the digestive system. It contains electrolytes and offers a subtle, refreshing taste to your smoothies.

Celery: Celery is composed mainly of water and contains electrolytes like potassium and sodium. It adds a mild flavour to your smoothies while contributing to hydration and electrolyte balance.

Herbal Infusions: Herbal infusions, such as hibiscus or mint tea, can be a hydrating base for your smoothies. They not only provide flavour but also offer additional health benefits and electrolytes.

Sea Salt: A pinch of sea salt in your smoothie can help replenish sodium, an important electrolyte lost through sweat during exercise. However, it's essential to use sea salt in moderation, as excessive sodium intake can have negative health effects.

CHAPTER SIX

Indulgent and Healthy Dessert Smoothies

Guilt-Free Sweet Treats

When it comes to weight loss, it's natural to have cravings for sweet treats. The good news is that you can satisfy those cravings guilt-free by incorporating wholesome ingredients into your weight loss smoothies. These guilt-free sweet treats are not only delicious but also packed with nutrients that support your weight loss goals. Here are some ideas for creating guilt-free sweet treats in the form of weight loss smoothies:

Banana and Peanut Butter Delight: Blend together a ripe banana, a tablespoon of natural peanut butter, a cup of unsweetened almond milk, and a sprinkle of cinnamon. This creamy and satisfying smoothie offers a combination of natural sweetness, healthy fats, and protein.

Berry Blast: Combine a cup of mixed berries (such as strawberries, blueberries, and raspberries), a scoop of vanilla protein powder, a handful of spinach, and water or unsweetened almond milk. This refreshing smoothie is packed with antioxidants, vitamins, and fibre.

Green Apple Pie: Blend together a green apple (cored and sliced), a scoop of vanilla protein powder, a handful of spinach, a dash of cinnamon, a tablespoon of almond butter, and water or unsweetened almond milk. This smoothie gives you the taste of apple pie while offering fibre, vitamins, and a touch of sweetness.

Decadent Flavours with Nutritional Benefits

Who says weight loss smoothies have to be bland and boring? With a little creativity, you can create smoothies that are not only decadently flavorful but also packed with nutritional benefits to support your weight loss journey. Here are some ideas for incorporating decadent flavours into your weight loss smoothies while still reaping the benefits of wholesome ingredients:

Chocolate Delight: Use unsweetened cocoa powder or cacao powder to add a rich chocolate flavour to your smoothies. Cocoa powder is a good source of antioxidants and can contribute to a satisfying and indulgent experience.

Coffee Kick: Add a shot of espresso or a teaspoon of instant coffee to your smoothie for a delightful mocha flavour. Coffee can provide a natural energy boost and may even help increase metabolism.

Nutty Goodness: Incorporate a tablespoon of nut butter, such as almond butter or cashew butter, into your smoothie for a creamy and nutty taste. Nut butters offer healthy fats, protein, and fibre, keeping you feeling satisfied and providing essential nutrients.

Citrus Zest: Add a squeeze of lemon or lime juice, or zest from their peels, to your smoothie for a burst of citrus flavour. Citrus fruits are rich in vitamin C and can help enhance the flavour of other fruits in the blend.

CHAPTER SEVEN

Incorporating Superfoods into Your Smoothies

Understanding the Power of Superfoods

Superfoods are nutrient-dense ingredients that offer exceptional health benefits. Incorporating superfoods into your weight loss smoothies can enhance their nutritional value and support your weight loss goals. Here's a closer look at the power of superfoods and how they can be beneficial in weight loss smoothies:

Nutrient Density: Superfoods are packed with essential vitamins, minerals, and antioxidants. They offer a concentrated dose of nutrients in every serving, making them a valuable addition to weight loss smoothies. Nutrient-dense ingredients support overall health, boost immunity, and provide the necessary fuel for your body to function optimally.

Antioxidant-Rich: Many superfoods are known for their high antioxidant content. Antioxidants help combat oxidative stress and protect the body against free radicals, which can contribute to inflammation and various health conditions. By incorporating antioxidant-rich superfoods like berries, dark leafy greens, or cacao powder into your smoothies, you support cellular health and overall well-being.

Fibre Content: Superfoods are often excellent sources of dietary fibre. By including fibre-rich superfoods like chia seeds, flaxseeds, or oats in your smoothies, you can feel fuller for longer and support healthy digestion, which can contribute to weight loss.

Metabolism Boosters: Certain superfoods have properties that can boost metabolism and increase calorie burning. Ingredients like green tea, cayenne pepper, or ginger have thermogenic effects, meaning they can increase the body's calorie expenditure and support weight loss efforts. Incorporating these metabolism-boosting superfoods into your smoothies can give your weight loss journey an extra kick.

Blood Sugar Regulation: Superfoods that are low on the glycemic index, such as leafy greens, cruciferous vegetables, or cinnamon, can help regulate blood sugar levels. Stable blood sugar levels are crucial for weight management, as they prevent energy crashes, reduce cravings, and support balanced insulin levels. Including these blood sugar-regulating superfoods in your smoothies can help keep your energy levels stable throughout the day.

Adaptogens: Some superfoods, known as adaptogens, have unique properties that help the body adapt to stress and promote balance. Adaptogens like ashwagandha, maca, or holy basil can support adrenal health and assist in managing stress-related weight gain. Adding adaptogenic superfoods to your smoothies can help regulate cortisol levels and support overall well-being.

CHAPTER EIGHT

Boosting Your Weight Loss Journey with Lifestyle Changes

While weight loss smoothies can be a valuable addition to your weight loss journey, it's important to remember that sustainable and long-term weight loss is best achieved through a holistic approach that includes lifestyle changes. Here are some lifestyle changes that can complement the use of weight loss smoothies and boost your overall weight loss journey:

Balanced Diet: Alongside weight loss smoothies, focus on consuming a balanced diet that includes a variety of nutrient-dense foods. Include whole grains, fruits, vegetables, lean proteins, and healthy fats in your meals. Opt for whole, unprocessed foods whenever possible and practice portion control to create a calorie deficit necessary for weight loss.

Regular Exercise: Engaging in regular physical activity is crucial for weight loss and overall health. Combine your weight loss smoothie regimen with a well-rounded exercise routine that includes cardiovascular exercises, strength training, and flexibility exercises. Aim for at least 150 minutes of moderate-intensity aerobic activity or 75 minutes of vigorous-intensity aerobic activity per week, along with strength training exercises at least two days a week.

Hydration: Staying hydrated is essential for overall health and can also support weight loss. Drink an adequate amount of water throughout the day to keep your body hydrated and promote proper digestion. Water can also help control appetite and reduce calorie intake, making it a valuable ally in your weight loss journey.

Portion Control: While weight loss smoothies can be nutritious and filling, it's important to practise portion control with all your meals and snacks. Consider your portion proportions and try not to overeat. To help you manage portion sizes and pay attention to your body's hunger and fullness cues, think about utilising smaller plates and bowls.

Mindful Eating: Adopting mindful eating practices can help you develop a healthier relationship with food. Know your body's hunger and fullness signals, eat slowly, and savour each bite. Avoid distractions during meals, such as screens or multitasking, and focus on the sensory experience of eating. This can help prevent overeating and promote mindful food choices.

Stress Management: Chronic stress can hinder weight loss progress. Implement stress management techniques like meditation, deep breathing exercises, yoga, or engaging in hobbies and activities that bring you joy. Managing stress effectively can help prevent emotional eating and support a healthier mindset towards weight loss.

Quality Sleep: Prioritise getting adequate sleep each night as it plays a crucial role in weight management. Hormones that control appetite can be disturbed by sleep deprivation, which can increase desires and cause overeating. To help your efforts to lose weight, aim for 7-9 hours of good sleep each night.

Exercise and Physical Activity Recommendations

Exercise and physical activity play a vital role in achieving weight loss and overall health. When combined with weight loss smoothies, they can help maximise your results and support a sustainable weight loss journey. Here are some exercise and physical activity recommendations to complement your weight loss smoothie regimen:

Cardiovascular Exercise: Engage in regular cardiovascular exercises to burn calories and increase your heart rate. This includes activities like brisk walking, jogging, cycling, swimming, dancing, or using cardio machines at the gym. Aim for at least 150 minutes of moderate-intensity aerobic activity or 75 minutes of vigorous-intensity aerobic activity per week. Spread your sessions throughout the week to ensure consistency.

Strength Training: Incorporate strength training exercises to build lean muscle mass. Strength training not only helps tone and define your muscles but also boosts your metabolism, allowing you to burn more calories even at rest. Include exercises that target major muscle groups, such as squats, lunges, push-ups, and dumbbell or resistance band exercises. Aim for at least two days of strength training per week, allowing a day of rest between sessions.

High-Intensity Interval Training (HIIT): Consider adding HIIT workouts to your exercise routine. HIIT involves alternating between intense bursts of exercise and short recovery periods. This type of training is effective for burning calories, increasing cardiovascular fitness, and improving metabolic rate. HIIT workouts can be performed with various exercises such as sprints, jumping jacks, burpees, or bodyweight exercises. Start with shorter intervals and gradually increase the intensity and duration as your fitness level improves.

Flexibility and Stretching: Don't forget to include flexibility exercises to improve your range of motion and prevent injuries. Incorporate stretching, yoga, or Pilates into your routine to increase flexibility, improve posture, and promote relaxation. Stretching after workouts can help reduce muscle soreness and improve recovery.

Consistency and Progression: Consistency is key when it comes to exercise. Aim to make physical activity a regular part of your routine by scheduling workouts and sticking to them. Gradually increase the duration, intensity, or frequency of your workouts over time to challenge your body and continue making progress.

Stress Management and Sleep Optimization

Stress management and quality sleep are essential components of a successful weight loss journey. When combined with weight loss smoothies, they can further enhance your results and support overall well-being. Here are some strategies for stress management and sleep optimization to complement your weight loss smoothie regimen:

Mindfulness and Meditation: Practise mindfulness techniques such as deep breathing exercises, meditation, or guided imagery. These practices can help reduce stress, improve focus, and promote a sense of calm. Dedicate a few minutes each day to mindfulness exercises to help manage stress levels.

Physical Activity: Engage in regular physical activity, as exercise can help reduce stress and release endorphins, which improve mood. Choose activities you enjoy, such as walking, yoga, or dancing, and make them a part of your routine.

Time Management: Prioritise tasks and set realistic goals to avoid feeling overwhelmed. Break large tasks into smaller, manageable steps, and allocate time for self-care activities and relaxation.

Consistent Sleep Schedule: Establish a regular sleep schedule by going to bed and waking up at the same time each day, even on weekends. This helps regulate your body's internal clock and promotes better sleep quality.

Create a Relaxing Sleep Environment: Make your bedroom a calm and comfortable sleep environment. Ensure your room is dark, quiet, and at a comfortable temperature. Remove distractions such as electronics and consider using earplugs, eye masks, or white noise machines if needed.

Limit Stimulants and Electronic Devices: Avoid consuming caffeine or stimulants close to bedtime, as they can interfere with sleep. Additionally, limit exposure to electronic devices (e.g., smartphones, tablets, computers) before bed, as the blue light emitted can disrupt sleep patterns.

Create a Relaxing Bedtime Ritual: Incorporate a soothing activity into your bedtime routine, such as sipping a cup of herbal tea, practising gentle stretching or relaxation exercises, or journaling to release any lingering thoughts or worries.

Sustainable Habits for Long-Term Success

Weight loss smoothies can be a valuable tool in your weight loss journey, but to achieve long-term success, it's important to adopt sustainable habits that support a healthy lifestyle. Here are some sustainable habits to incorporate alongside weight loss smoothies for long-term success:

Mindful Eating: Practise mindful eating by paying attention to your body's hunger and fullness cues. Eat slowly, savour each bite, and be aware of the taste, texture, and satisfaction of your meals. Avoid distractions while eating, such as screens or multitasking, and focus on the experience of nourishing your body.

Portion Control: To practise portion control you have to be mindful of portion sizes. Use measuring cups, a food scale, or other portion-control tools to ensure you're consuming appropriate serving sizes. Over time, your perception of portion sizes will improve, making it easier to maintain a balanced diet.

Balanced Nutrition: Ensure that your weight loss smoothies are balanced in terms of macronutrients and include a variety of fruits, vegetables, proteins, healthy fats, and fibre. Incorporate whole, unprocessed foods into your meals to provide essential nutrients and promote overall health.

Regular Physical Activity: Engage in regular physical activity that you enjoy and that fits into your lifestyle. Find activities that you can incorporate into your daily routine, such as walking, cycling, swimming, or group fitness classes. Aim for a combination of cardiovascular exercises, strength training, and flexibility exercises for a well-rounded fitness routine.

Regular Self-Reflection: Take time to reflect on your progress, challenges, and successes. Celebrate your achievements, learn from setbacks, and make adjustments as needed. Regular self-reflection helps you stay motivated and committed to your weight loss goals.

Support System: Surround yourself with a supportive network of friends, family, or even online communities that share similar goals. Seek support, accountability, and encouragement from others on your weight loss journey.

CONCLUSION

In conclusion, weight loss smoothies can be a delicious and nutritious addition to your weight loss journey. They offer a convenient and versatile way to incorporate a variety of ingredients that support your health and weight loss goals. By selecting the right ingredients, blending techniques, and incorporating them into your daily routine, you can experience the benefits of weight loss smoothies.

Throughout this guide, we explored various aspects of weight loss smoothies, from understanding macronutrients and choosing the right ingredients to optimising nutrition and addressing specific needs such as muscle recovery, hydration, and cravings. We also discussed the importance of incorporating other lifestyle factors such as exercise, stress management, sleep, and sustainable habits for long-term success.

Always consult with a healthcare professional or registered dietitian before making significant changes to your diet or exercise routine, especially if you have any underlying health conditions or dietary restrictions.

By incorporating weight loss smoothies into your lifestyle and adopting healthy habits, you can achieve your weight loss goals while enjoying the benefits of improved nutrition, increased energy levels, and enhanced vitality. Cheers to your success and a healthier, happier you.